Acne:
How to get rid of acne - scientifically

James Hughes BA (Hons), PG Dip., MA

CONTENTS

PREFACE

I let my skin beat me for 20 years.

My acne held me back. It stopped me enjoying life – and caused me to limit my own career and aspirations.

There were jobs I didn't apply for, even though I was well qualified. There were nights I couldn't face going out with friends because of a fresh eruption. There were girls I didn't ask out.

My well-meaning friends and family made suggestions about what I could do. Some were old wives' tales, some were based on dodgy websites, occasionally it was even based on science.

And I hated those conversations, because I hated talking about my spots.

Every time a new treatment came out I would go straight to the store to buy it. I would even try treatments available in other countries in case they were the silver bullet.

I spent thousands of pounds every year importing them – and meeting unexpected customs charges.

I tried everything.

I went from anger to despair to gradual acceptance. And that last stage was the worst – because I gave up.

I went about my skincare routine – the best I had managed to come up with – and stuck to it. But it was about managing the spots rather than curing them once and for all.

But then I decided to take back control – and I hope that buying this book is your first step to doing the same.

I read everything I could. I spoke to doctors and to dermatologists. I questioned what they were telling me and did my own research.

This book is the result of that research. It is the book I wish I had been given 20 years ago.

I hope it works for you.

Don't despair. And don't give up.

There is an answer for you out there – and the chances are it is in here.

Here is the thing about acne. There isn't enough science. Some people say one thing – some people say another.

For a condition that millions of people suffer from daily there is very little time or money being spent solving it.

Why? Because acne, more than virtually any other condition, is individual.

It means that what works for a friend or another member of the family may not work for you.

That is why I have tried to include as many options as possible for you here.

There is no miracle cure, no matter what some books would have you believe (trust me – been there, done that, spent the money, suffered the disappointment).

What you must do is work through the options – and stick with each long enough to give your skin time to react.

(Hint – that is more than a week.)

Start getting scientific about this. The worst case scenario, after all, is discovering the combination of treatments that works for you... and not being able to remember what it was.

When you reach the end of the road (or the end of your patience) don't be afraid to go to your doctor.

I put it off because I thought I would be wasting their time.

When I eventually plucked up courage, I was given treatments that didn't work for my particular sort of acne.

And I gave up. I didn't go back because I didn't realise that there were other treatments that the doctor could prescribe.

This book will tell you what they are – and the pros and cons of each.

So, work through this book. If something doesn't work for you, draw a line through it and move on.

You're a step nearer solving your acne problem than you would have been if you haven't tried it.

But, if you are like me you won't want to wait.

Being scientific sounds sensible. But it also sounds slow.

What I want to do is give you the best of both worlds.

This book will list the treatments – the things to try – while also giving you hints and tips that you can start using right now, today.

That includes 12 ways you might actually be making your acne worse without realizing.

After my conversations with doctors, dermatologists and makeup artists I badly want to go back in time and tell myself that some of the stuff I was convinced would help - was actually doing the exact opposite.

(By the way – after reading it, I promise that you will never look at your phone in the same way again!)

So feel free to skip through to the sections of the book that you will find most helpful – grab some quick cheats to help see you through until your acne is nailed for good.

But, please, whatever you do – avoid the one mistake that most people make about their spots.

And that is just seeing them as "spots" or "zits".

Acne is a catch-all term that covers a whole range of different conditions.

It's another reason why some treatments that work well for one person just don't seem to have any impact for someone else (or might even make things worse).

Take a moment to read through and identify exactly what you have – and how bad it is. Because once you've done that you will be in a far stronger position to know what might fix it.

And here is my one last piece of advice as an acne survivor before we begin the book proper.

Please – if nothing else, remember this.

Your acne is temporary. Out there (or, hopefully, in here!) there is a solution that will help you.

But once that acne is gone for good don't find yourself stuck with scarring. That is far more likely to last longer than the spots ever did.

So, as much as you sometimes want to physically rip that acne off your face – don't squeeze or pop or scratch.

It's storing up trouble for you that will last decades after your spots have finally gone for good.

1
INTRODUCTION

Acne is an immensely common skin condition that affects people of all ages and has a broad range of levels in regards to severity. The scientific term for acne is acne vulgaris, which literally means, "common acne." There has been a significant amount of controversy as to the exact cause of acne. For instance, dermatologists once claimed that eating greasy foods and chocolate was to blame for pimples. Is that true? Well, we try to get to grips with the truth later in this book.

Acne is a chronic skin condition that affects most people at some point during their life. It causes spots to develop on the skin, usually on the face, back and chest. The symptoms of acne can be mild, moderate or severe.

Acne is thought to be caused by changes in hormones that are triggered during puberty.

Acne can cause great distress and have an adverse effect on a person's quality of life and self-esteem.

So healthcare professionals recognise that the condition requires effective and sometimes aggressive treatment.

And, if you've got it, that's actually good news. It means you won't have to convince anyone to take you seriously.

How common is acne?

If you want to skip straight to the treatments – then be my guest.

But this might reassure you that you aren't alone.

Acne is the most common type of skin condition. It is most widespread among older children, teenagers and young adults.

Around 80% of 11 to 30-year-olds are affected by acne. Most acne cases in girls occur between the ages of 14 to 17, and in boys the condition is most common in 16 to 19-year-olds.

Most people will experience repeated episodes, or flare-ups, of acne for several years before finding that their symptoms gradually start to improve as they get older. The symptoms of acne usually disappear when a person is in their twenties.

However, in some cases, acne can continue into adult life, with approximately 5% of women and 1% of men over 25 continuing to experience symptoms.

Acne is a skin disease that is characterized by the appearance of pimples on various parts of the body such as the neck, face, back, chest as well as shoulders. The disease, which is very common, is a result of clogged up hair follicles caused by oil and dead skin cells. For most people who suffer from acne it is an embarrassing problem that does not easily go away, even after treatment has been administered.

Sometimes the pimples might disappear only to reappear again after a certain time period if the treatment used is not effective. The symptoms of acne are varied. The common appearances are (tender) red bumps, pustules, cysts and congested pores which are commonly referred to as black or white heads.

More recent research has suggested that hormonal fluctuation in the body may be the main cause of acne, such as during puberty, pregnancy, menstruation, and times of stress when the skin tends to be more oily. When dead skin cells and sebum (the natural oil produced by glands in the skin) clog pores, acne forms and can become quite severe if left untreated. Fortunately, there are various treatment methods, from facial cleansers with benzoyl peroxide or salicylic acid, to natural remedies like tea-tree oil and apple cider vinegar. Some of them are more effective than others and some will be effective for some people and not to others. It depends of what kind of acne you have.

Stick with this book – and we'll tell you what the options are and how to work through them.

Dermatologists generally recommend to begin treating acne with a daily skin care regimen before utilizing the more extreme or hazardous modes of treatment, such as laser therapy or dermabrasion. A daily skin care regimen is essential for preventing and treating acne, as well as maintaining a proper balance of oil within the skin. Acne begins forming about 90 days before it actually appears above the surface of the skin, which means that even during times when no acne can be seen, a daily skin care regimen should still be strictly adhered to. An example of a basic skin care routine is as follows:

Choose a mild facial cleanser depending on the severity of acne and wash in the morning and at night.

After each wash, pat dry and apply a toner or astringent to the entire face with a cotton ball and let dry.

Apply an acne medication cream or gel directly to any pimples or the entire face if needed.

If dryness becomes a problem after a few days, begin applying an oil-free moisturizer as a fourth step.

For body acne, choose an exfoliating acne body wash and implement during every shower or bath.

Not all acne products are created equal, and each person reacts differently to certain acne medications, which means it may take some trial and error for an individual to locate an effective acne treatment. In addition, it can take upwards of a few weeks to a month before substantial results are experienced. After such treatment has been tried and failed, it may be time to make an appointment with a dermatologist who can devise an acne treatment specifically tailored for each patient.

Acne involves a disorder with glands in the skin that are located next to hair follicles. These glands, called sebaceous glands, secrete an oily substance called sebum. Everyone has these glands, and the secretion of sebum is normal, but people with acne have larger glands that release more sebum in into the skin. The excess sebum can trap oil, bacteria, and skin cells. One bacterium in particular, known as P. acnes, is able to thrive in these conditions. P. acnes is normally present in the skin, however in people with acne they are present in much greater numbers. The growth and proliferation of these bacteria can cause inflammation of the skin, leading to pimples.

Diagnosis

In most cases, a dermatologist or other healthcare provider can diagnose by examining the affected skin. However, your doctor may ask several questions that are aimed at ensuring a proper acne diagnosis and to rule out other skin disorders. These include questions about:

Areas of sensitive skin, or eczema

Other diseases that may affect the ability to handle medications

Previous drug allergies

Use of steroids (for bodybuilding, for example)

Mood disorders or depression

Use of contraceptives, irregular menstrual period, current or past pregnancy, breast feeding

In some cases acne can mimic other related skin disorders, such as rosacea. This information will help your doctor make an informed diagnosis.

Emotional Consequences

Having acne does not just mean superficial or cosmetic changes to the skin—it has an emotional aspect to it as well. Since the face is one of the primary areas affected by acne, symptoms of the disease can change the appearance of those affected, and this can lead to stress and anxiety. Depending on the severity of the condition, acne can lead to a negative self-image, including:

Low self-esteem

Loss of confidence

Depression

2
WHAT'S CAUSING YOUR ACNE

Acne is a disorder that is caused by the sebaceous gland of the skin. This gland is more commonly known as the hair follicle. The skin is covered with these tiny openings. The only exceptions to this are the bottom of the feet, the palms of the hand, the top of the feet, and the lower part of the lips. The chest, upper part of the neck, and the face are the parts of the body with the most sebaceous glands on them. This is what causes acne to be more common in these areas.

Sebum is secreted by the sebaceous glands. This substance is what is responsible for the hair and skin staying soft and moisturized. When you are in your teens or pubescent years, these glands are larger than normal and the amount of sebum produced is being controlled by the large amounts of hormones in the body. Once you make it to around twenty years of age, the amount of secretion will begin to go down as the hormone levels regulate themselves.

There is a bacterial substance on the skin that is medically known as Propionic bacterium acnes. This is what causes acne. This bacteria grows and thrives on the sebum. During the years of puberty, the propionic bacterium acnes bacteria are at their highest level, because the sebum level is also high. Individuals who have acne have an overgrowth of the bacteria in the sebaceous glands, compared to those who do not suffer from acne.

When the bacteria are present, white blood cells are also present in the gland. The white blood cells are damaging to the follicle wall and this brings the sebum and bacteria into the dermis layer of the skin. The bacteria can also activate the fatty acids in the body and cause further irritation to the gland. The gland swells from this activity and what causes acne to appear.

Normal glands will produce sebum that will join with exfoliating cells of the skin and this will make the gland full. The gland then lets these ingredients out, causing the face to feel oily. If nothing is in the way to hinder this process, the skin stays in balance with the correct moisture it needs and stays strong and healthy. When the sebum and cells in the gland are not able to come out as they should, the skin gets dry in spots and the result of the clogged gland is a blackhead or whitehead. And here is the kicker – there is no known reason for it.

Anyone in the world can suffer with acne. It does not matter where you are from or what age you are. It doesn't matter if you are rich, poor, male or female - it can still affect you. This is because everyone's skin is different. We all have various factors that cause our own forms of acne.

The first thing you need to do so you can start to treat your acne is to find out what type of skin you have. This is so you can decide on the most effective course for treatment. For example if you have oily skin you do not want to be using moisturizing products, cosmetics or cleansing products that are oil based.

You need to be purchasing products that are oil free. Using the same logic, if you have dry skin you need to be using oil based products because you skin needs the extra oil.

All types of skin need to be moisturized every day, even oily skin. There are a lot of good, oil free moisturizers available for use on oily skin. Dry skin, however, comes with its own set of problems and moisturizing should be done with a product specifically designed for dry skin.

Prescription medication in the form of ointments and creams is available via your doctor and they will help keep your breakouts dry and can even help speed up cell replacement in the acne infected areas of your skin. Topical treatments (that you rub on your skin) are designed to stop the pores clogging while they remove excess dirt and oil from the skin's surface, at the same time removing any acne causing bacteria. There are also natural remedies available that claim to be able to help with the treatment of acne.

Before you start to understand your acne problem you need to look at what causes it. Understanding the cause will help you in developing the proper treatment for your acne.

Take a look at these triggers...

Stress - This plays a big role in the development of your acne. The body releases chemicals and hormones that turn into toxins and waste when it becomes tense and needs to expel them. Some of these end up being expelled through the skin and this helps contribute towards your acne problem.

Hormones - The early teenage years bring many changes to the body and these changes often cause repeated breakouts of pustules, pimples and even cysts (all defined later in the book). The adult years are no different, especially for women. Premenstrual and menopausal problems can cause acne problems for a lot of women. Hormone related acne produces extra oil, so products that help to reduce or eliminate oil will be the best for this type of acne.

Skin care products and cosmetics - It is important to choose the right products for your skin. Using the incorrect product will contribute to your acne. Using oily products on oily skin will only make it worse, so you must check that the products match your skin type.

Chocolate - There are those that still believe that chocolate and sweets are a contributing factor to acne. The subject is still widely researched and debated. A lot of experts say that it has nothing to do with acne, but they cannot be 100% certain.

The lifestyle you live and the environment you live in are both contributing factors to what causes your acne problems. You need to learn how to take care of your skin, keep it moisturized, hydrated and learn how to reduce the factors that will cause your acne attacks.

Steroids and Specific Medications - It is wise to stop overusing vitamins. Even if one "miracle cure" advises the exact opposite (I tried it. Didn't work). Vitamins are essential to our skin but overusing them can actually cause acne. Examples include B1, B6 and B12. Abuse or inappropriate use of steroids, especially anabolic steroids can lead to acne breakouts because they stimulate sebaceous glands.

Harsh and Rough Cleansing – It's tempting to try to scrub the acne away – to be so angry you just want to get it off your face, even though you know it's doing you damage. This kind of cleansing can damage the skin layers and spread infections. So, be gentle (even if you don't want to be). When cleansing your skin, use lukewarm water. Water that is too hot can dehydrate your skin and too cold can dry it out.

Picking or squeezing and the environment - High humidity causes the skin to swell and pollution in the environment can cause clogging of your pores. Avoid picking and s□ueezing pimples or acne outbreaks as this can send infections deeper into the skin and cause scarring.

Your genes - As I said earlier, some causes of acne are inevitable. This is a good example of a cause of acne that you just can't avoid. Acne can be inherited and some types, such as cystic acne can come from family members such as parents or grandparents.

Extra Sebum in the Follicle - When hormones stimulate your sebaceous glands, they produces extra sebum, which mixes with dead skin cells and skin bacteria. This is a normal process, but excess sebum in the follicle increases the chances of clogging and acne. There are things that can lead to production of excess sebum like anabolic steroids.

So these are the common causes of acne breakouts. The best way to minimize acne breakouts is to take care of your body. There are popular products that can treat acne but some of them are not as effective as others.

If you have never had serious acne and all over a sudden you do, then it is best to find out what caused it. You may be dealing with something minor that you can take care of to get rid of your acne instead of just managing it.

3
TYPES OF ACNE
WHICH ONE DO YOU HAVE?

There are a range of different types of acne, ranging from mild to severe forms, with different causes and treatments. Knowing which type you have will help you deal with the problem most effectively.

Types of acne include:

Acne vulgaris (mild to moderate)

Acne vulgaris (moderate to severe)

Acne Rosacea

Acne Conglobata

Acne Fulminans

Gram negative folliculitis

Pyoderma Faciale

Acne Vulgaris (mild to moderate)
This is the most common form of acne. It usually consists of skin lesions such as whiteheads, blackheads, papules and pustules.

Whiteheads are caused by a follicle or pore becoming completely blocked with shed skin cells and oil or sebum accumulating behind the blockage, leading to the raised white appearance.

Blackheads result from partial blockage of a pore with slow leakage of trapped oil, bacteria and skin cells onto the skin surface. The characteristic dark colour is caused by the oxidation of skin pigment, melanin, on exposure to oxygen in the air at the skin's surface. Blackheads tend to be more stable than white heads and may take a long time to resolve.

Papules are inflamed, red, tender, raised areas that, in contrast to white heads or blackheads, do not have a 'core' or head.

Pustules appear generally similar to whiteheads except that they are more inflamed and red and the centre may appear more yellowed. This is a result of the bodies inflammatory immune reaction to the trapped oil and bacteria leading accumulation of white blood cells and leakage of fluid from capillaries.

Acne Vulgaris (moderate to severe)

Moderate to severe acne vulgaris is defined by the presence of nodules and cysts.

Nodules are large, firm, raised inflamed areas that, in contrast to the milder lesions mentioned above, are more deeply situated in the skin. These nodules can be quite painful and sometimes will last for a number of months.

A cyst is similar to a pustule but is larger (greater than 5mm in diametre) and more deeply seated within the skin. The cyst is full of pus, which is debris of bacteria, skin cells, and immune cells. These lesions are often painful and squeezing or trying to pop them can make this much worse by causing the accumulated pus to spread into surrounding tissues, widening the inflammatory reaction.

Acne Rosacea

Rosacea is characterized by a red rash, mostly on the nose, cheeks, chin and forehead. They are often associated white heads, bumps, blemishes and blood vessels (capillaries) may become more prominent.

In contrast to acne vulgaris, rosacea is more common in women and in people over 30 year of age.

Rosacea, if untreated over the long term may cause a condition called Rhinophyma. Rhinophyma is where there is excessive growth of the tissue affected by rosacea, which can lead to an enlarged and bumpy or knobby nose.

Treatments for rosacea differ to those for acne vulgaris so it is important that your doctor correctly identifies your condition.

Acne Conglobata

Acne conglobata is a rare, but particularly severe form of acne vulgaris that is most common in men aged 18-30 years old.

It consists of many large and often interconnected lesions that may spread across the face, back, buttock, upper arms, neck and chest.

Numerous blackheads are common. Unfortunately this type of acne is likely to lead to scarring, which in severe cases may be permanently disfiguring.

Treatment is best guided by a specialist dermatologist and will often include isotretinoin.

Acne Fulminans

As the name suggests, acne fulminans is the sudden onset of severe acne, with nodular and cystic lesions similar to those seen in acne conglobata.

The lesions may progess to ulceration, which is the breakdown of the skin overlying the cysts or nodules. In addition, people with acne fulminans will feel generally unwell with fevers and arthralgias (aching of the joints).

This type of acne is most common in young men. Treatment will usually include isotretinoin and oral steroids such as prednisone. In contrast to some other types of acne, acne fulminans tends not to respond well to antibiotics.

Gram Negative Folliculitis

Gram negative folliculitis is a bacterial infection that results in cysts and pustules.

Sometimes this can be a complication of antibiotic treatment for other types of acne but fortunately it is quite uncommon. Treatment with isotretinoin is usually effective.

Pyoderma Faciale

Pyoderma faciale is a severe form of acne that occurs only in women, most often between 20-40 years of age.

This condition usually begins quite suddenly and can affect people who have never had acne of any type before. It will often resolve within a year but the nodules and pustules can cause permanent scarring.

4
THE SIGNS AND SYMPTOMS OF ACNE YOU NEED TO KNOW ABOUT

Acne is a huge term and the signs and symptoms of acne usually come in four forms - pustules, blackheads, whiteheads, and cysts. Pustules being the inflammatory form, and blackheads and whiteheads the non-inflammatory form.

People suffering this condition normally have oily skin with large pores. This particular condition is the result of excessive production of the natural oil called sebum that keeps the skin lubricated and moisturized.

Pustules, also commonly known as pimples or zits, are red in color, inflamed, and swell up. They occur due to the walls of hair follicles rupturing for some reason. When the rupture happens, the dead skin cells, sebum and bacteria will move down from the skin surface causing irritation that will soon result to inflammation. This inflammation will lead to the formation of pustules.

Blackheads are formed when the skin pores that are clogged are closer to the surface of the skin. This form of acne does not usually cause inflammation and so they do not develop into pimples. People used to think that the blackheads were caused by dirt that would go away if you washed more. You might still get told this. Ignore it. It's rubbish.

Being close to the skin surface, the melanin (the pigment in our skin that provides its color) on the clogged pores is oxidized resulting to the black coloration. Thus, it cannot be washed away by water and soap and it is not true that these are cause by dirt and poor skin hygiene.

On the other hand, whiteheads are more likely to be inflamed and develop into pimples. Unlike the blackheads, these are formed when the skin pores are clogged in deeper part of skin, and the lack of exit point will lead to whiteheads forming.

Another signs and symptoms of acne are cysts. These are larger than pimples but also red and inflamed. They form an inflamed, closed sac beneath the skin, and may contain fluid or semisolid substances.

These symptoms signify a more serious type of skin condition.

The signs and symptoms illustrated above are caused by excessive oil production by our sebaceous glands and skin pores that are clogged by dead skin cells. And the skin that undergoes this condition is typically oily and has large skin pores.

The symptoms of acne are more likely to occur in the areas of the skin where there are many oil glands. For instance, there are approximately 2,000 sebaceous glands in the forehead alone.

The face, chest, shoulders and back have more areas that contain high number of these glands.

5
12 WAYS YOU MAY BE MAKING YOUR ACNE WORSE

You may think you're doing everything you can to treat your acne. But little things could add up to make it worse. Do any of these mistakes sound familiar?

Your cell phone is dirty

Think about it: your face produces oil and sweat, which gets onto your phone when you're on a call.

If you don't clean that off, during your next call you're pushing it back into your skin, along with any bacteria that has grown.

To clean it, follow the instructions from your phone's maker. You might try ear buds or another hands-free headset. Pressure from holding your phone against your cheek can also cause breakouts by irritating your skin.

You put your hair products too close to your hairline

If you use an anti-frizz product, or a thick gel or pomade, apply it away from your forehead.

Otherwise, you can get a line of acne right there at your hair line.

You quit too soon

"Everyone wants clear skin yesterday, but we have no silver bullet that works immediately. Acne treatments take weeks to start kicking in," says dermatologist Joshua Zeichner, MD, of Mt. Sinai Hospital in New York, who specializes in treating acne.

If over-the-counter acne products don't help within 2 to 4 weeks, then you may need to see a dermatologist. This is especially important if you have acne cysts or if your acne leaves scars.

You wash your face too much

"One of the biggest myths is: 'My face is dirty, and that's why I'm getting acne,'" says dermatologist Whitney Bowe, MD, of Advanced Dermatology P.C. in Westchester, N.Y.

"Washing too much can strip the skin of essential oils, leading the body to paradoxically produce more oil, which can lead to more pimples," Dr Zeichner adds.

Experts say washing twice a day is all you need.

You make mistakes when you wash your face

Don't use a dirty or damp washcloth when you wash. Bacteria can easily build up on them. Use a clean washcloth each time. I know it sounds crazy. After all – it's being washed when you put it into the sink, right? Wrong. You're getting it covered in oil and bacteria and then leaving them to breed on the side in the bathroom.

Also, don't exfoliate too often. Sandy or sugary products, rough scrubbing pads or loofahs, and even electric brushes can cause tiny tears in the skin if used daily. The result is irritation and inflammation.

That can make treating acne trickier. Exfoliate only once or twice a week

You pick and pop pimples

It's understandable to want to get rid of acne ASAP. But this particular plan of attack can cause deeper problems.

Instead of clearing the blockage out, you're pushing it further down - and that can lead to scarring.

Eating too many sweets or starchy foods

"When Mom told you to stay away from those items, she may have been on to something," Zeichner says.

No food is proven to cause acne. But sugary, processed ones such as white breads, white pasta, potato chips, cookies, and cakes may be linked to acne, says Bowe, who has researched this. There's no downside to limiting sugary foods.

Some studies have linked dairy products to acne, but that's not certain.

Not cleaning your makeup brushes and tools regularly

When did you last clean your makeup brush? Six months ago? Never? Everytime a professional makeup artist uses a brush on a client it gets washed.

There's a good reason – apart from getting rid of the color pigment.

Wouldn't it be gross if they kept spreading bacteria from face to face with dirty, gunky brushes? Not to mention that by contaminating makeup you are ultimately ruining it.

If you're not cleaning your own brushes at home at least weekly then you are asking for acne and potentially other nasties on your face.

Sleeping with makeup on

Why? Why? Why would you do this? Nothing about this is a good idea. Make-up professionals say that, even brands that claim not to clog your pores if left on overnight, should be removed before bed.

Sure, they might not clog your pores – but it will stop the skin renewing itself properly. Then you end up with bacteria build up and inflammation, which is what causes big pimples.

Yes, makeup remover wipes can be handy when you're just too tired to actually get to the sink and some soap, but this is not a good strategy for every day. If you just put in a little care into washing your face the right way you can actually make a world of difference in your skin.

This brings us to the importance of putting your face on clean things.

Not changing your pillow case and face towel often

Having clean pillowcases (especially if you've been sleeping with makeup on) and towels you use to dry off your face are super important.

You'll spend about 8 hours a night with your face on a pillow. If it's dirty, you are sleeping on dust and dead skin cells. How's that for gross?

Towels can also be lovely breeding grounds for bacteria, so think about what's touching your skin.

You use too much zit cream

This is what I like to call "pissing off your skin."

Everyone wants their acne to clear up quickly, so you may be tempted to slather on your treatment products several times (or more) per day. Over-using topical medications can't hurt, right? Besides, won't your acne clear up faster if you apply your medications more often.

You may be surprised to learn that applying too much medication, or applying too often, won't clear acne up any faster. But it will most definitely cause excessive drying, redness, peeling, and irritation.

In an effort to clear up skin, many people (I used to be one of them) will scrub excessively, morning and night with harsh or abrasive cleansers made for oily skin. This just dries out the skin, and doesn't actually deal with the root cause. In fact, it inflames the situation because the main cause of acne is an overproduction of sebum by sebaceous glands located at the root of hair follicles and using too many cleansing products cause your skin to produce more sebum, not less, creating an environment conducive to acne.

I know I'm preaching to the choir as I write this reminder that many ingredients in your beauty products are awful for your skin. These specifically include (but aren't limited to):

Mineral oil

Petrolatum

Lanolin

Perfume

Artificial colors

Alcohol

Only treating your skin from the outside

Your skin is a reflection of what's going on inside your body. So your acne could be from any combination of hormone imbalance, excess sebum production, stress, tobacco use, food allergies and high blood sugar from an unhealthy diet.

While it is helpful to properly treat your skin topically, real change as I've experienced it firsthand, comes from addressing the inner balance of the body in addition.

6
FIGHTING ACNE WITH FOOD

Can what you eat worsen or help your acne?

Acne is a multi-factorial disease. While each case is unique, you can greatly improve your chances of clear skin with food and lifestyle strategies.

Our skin is the largest organ in our body, and it's a complex ecosystem made up of several layers and components.

The skin is semi-permeable, meaning that although it's mostly a barrier between us and our environment, some stuff can get in and out. Sweat glands and hair follicles provide openings.

Hair originates in follicles deep in the subcutaneous layer, the deepest layer below the dermis. These hair follicles are paired with sebaceous glands, which secrete sebum, an oily substance that lubricates both hair and skin. It's why your hair gets greasy if you don't wash it. Human sebum is primarily composed of triglycerides (40-60%), cerides (19-26%), squalene (11-15%), and small amounts of cholesterol.

We have hair follicles and sebaceous glands all over our body, except for the palms of our hands and soles of our feet.

Acne forms when pores become congested with old skin cells, which is more likely when the skin is oily and skin cells stick together. If we also have high levels of bacteria on the skin plus systemic inflammation, we have ourselves a full-fledged acne party.

What contributes to acne?

Anything that clogs pores, and/or creates or worsens infection and inflammation, contributes. The major players in acne production are:

Excessive sebum (oil) production by the skin

Rapid division of skin cells

Delayed skin cell separation and death

Bacteria on the skin surface

Inflammatory response

The food we eat and our body fat cells play a role in sebum production, hormones, and inflammation. Hormonal changes likely have the greatest influence on acne (think birth control medications, anabolic steroids and puberty).

Hormonal factors

Growth hormone and IGF-1

Acne during puberty is often associated more with growth hormone (GH) than with testosterone and estrogens. GH goes from the brain to the liver and triggers the release of Insulin like Growth Factor-1 (IGF-1). IGF-1 promotes skin cell growth/division, sebum production, efficacy of luteinizing hormone (LH) and the production of estrogens.

Insulin and glycemic response

A study published in the *Canadian Medical Association Journal* in 1958 described acne as "diabetes of the skin." And as far as I'm concerned, everything from the 1950s was true... Ahem.

High insulin levels and insulin resistance are associated with worse acne and more sebum (side note: more body fat can lead to more insulin resistance). Medications that lower insulin and control glucose often have the side effect of less acne.

Androgens

Acne severity doesn't seem to correlate with total androgen levels in the body. Rather, androgens play a permissive role in priming or initiating acne. An example of this would be women with PCOS or someone starting a cycle of anabolic/androgenic steroids. These folks often experience a surge of circulating androgens and IGF-1, along with lower levels of sex hormone binding proteins.

Androgens can directly influence skin cells if the cells have high levels of androgen receptors. Also, androgens can increase growth and productivity of sebaceous glands.

Consuming a lot of food promotes androgen release in the body. Animal foods and saturated fats tend to get the biggest response. Lower fat, higher fiber diets can increase levels of sex hormone binding proteins, thus lowering free levels of circulating androgens.

Inflammation & stress

Acne is a type of inflammatory disease. With acne, inflammatory hormones and cell signals are unregulated — the skin is a hive of inflammatory activity.

Our bodies secrete cortisol in response to stress. Evidence shows that people with acne have an over-active cortisol secretion system, one that is particularly expressed in the sebaceous glands.

Thus, stress (whether physical or general life stress) plus inflammation (whether existing or prompted by stress) make acne worse.

Nutrition: What makes acne worse?
Not enough antioxidant vitamins and minerals

Low levels of vitamin C and E, zinc, selenium, and carotenoids might contribute to acne. These nutrients help fight free radicals that break down skin elastin, produce collagen, and repair skin damage. The catch here is that you usually have to get these from whole foods for them to be of any benefit.

Processed foods
Data show a mixed relationship between processed foods and acne. Eat a big meal with lots of processed food and you have lots of insulin. Lots of insulin means lots of tissue growth and androgen production, which are both contributors to acne.

Foods that are highly processed and cooked often contain compounds that promote oxidative stress and inflammation. Again, oxidative stress and inflammation almost always contribute to chronic disease.

Dairy
While there have been noted associations between dairy consumption and acne starting back in the 1800s, some data indicates no association. So that's useful...

Milk provides a mix of growth factors, hormones and nutrients specific to offspring. As rapid growth ends and the youngster can feed themselves, milk consumption is stopped (well, not in humans).

Dairy foods produce a high insulin response, increase hormone levels in the body and alter inflammation – all factors that lead to unfavorable acne outcomes.

Consuming cow's milk can raise IGF-1 levels 10-20% in the body. IGF-1 from cow's milk survives pasteurization and homogenization and digestion in our gut, and can enter the body as an intact hormone (cow and human IGF-1 share the same sequence).

The unfavorable associations between dairy and acne haven't been noticed with fermented dairy products, maybe because bacteria in fermented dairy use IGF-1, leaving less for us to absorb.

Some experts theorize that whey protein in particular may encourage acne, since it's a strong promoter of insulin. A compound called betacellulin (which can be found in dairy foods) may increase skin cell division and decrease skin cell death – leading to worse acne.

Alcohol

Many studies link alcohol consumption to acne.

GI dysfunction & gluten

Acne is often correlated with GI tract dysfunction.

Those with acne might be more likely to experience gastrointestinal problems like bloating and constipation.

Gut health is often diminished when chronically stressed, leading to inflammation and maybe even a leaky gut.

There may be a connection between wheat gluten and acne (as well as between gluten and other skin conditions). Consider eliminating all sources of wheat and gluten from your diet for a month and see if that helps.

Nutrition: What makes acne better?

Acne is a big deal. While genetics (mom seems to play a bigger role) and ethnicity contribute to acne, it appears that how we live each day matters too.

In the US, people spend more than $100 million on over-the-counter products to fight acne. Yet many non-Westernized populations have no acne at all.

So, you could spend a lot of money on drugs that have potentially dangerous side effects... or you could change your diet. Changing your diet is a lot cheaper and safer as a starting point. But don't rule out drugs. More on them to come.

Whole plant foods

Diets based around whole plants can lead to slightly lower IGF-1 levels and slightly higher IGF-1 binding protein levels (leaving less available IGF-1 circulating in the body). This might help reduce acne.

Not Overeating

Less food coming into the body is associated with less sebum production.

Phytoestrogens

These substances, found in foods such as soy, may inhibit androgen-forming and acne-promoting enzymes, but don't appear to play a major role in helping acne.

Cocoa

There doesn't seem to be an association between chocolate (in its most unprocessed form) and acne.

Studies show that dark chocolate can improve insulin sensitivity and improve blood flow to the skin and skin hydration.

Some manufacturers are even capitalizing on these studies by offering chocolate in skin products. The jury's still out on whether this works, but it sure makes you smell tasty.

Omega-3 fats

Skin levels of fatty acids might play a role in the development of acne.

Furthermore, the pro-inflammatory Western diet (with lots of omega-6 fats) tends to negatively influence acne.

Balancing fat intake and ensuring enough omega-3s seems to be important for overall skin health. 1 gram of EPA from a supplement (check your fish oil to see how much EPA is in it) might be useful for acne treatment.

GI health

As mentioned earlier, poor GI health is strongly correlated with acne. Whole foods, soluble and insoluble fibre, omega-3 fats, coconut, and Brassica vegetables (cauliflower, broccoli, Brussels sprouts, cabbage, kohlrabi, etc.) can have a beneficial influence on gut health, in part by improving gut motility.

Fibre can also bind to and excrete excess hormones that contribute to acne.

Consider eliminating wheat, dairy, and sugar for a month to see if this helps. All of these things worsen GI tract problems, and acne is strongly connected to gluten enteropathy.

Pre/Probiotics

This might be of particular interest to anyone who has been using antibiotics for acne.

Our gut is home to countless bacteria and if gut health is out of whack, this might have a negative influence on acne. Getting enough of these from foods and/or supplements can help to restore gut health and may reduce acne.

Skin cells have also been found to act as immune cells that signal an over-active immune system. Inflamed skin means inflamed body, and probably inflamed gut.

Spices

Many spices (eg cinnamon, ginger, turmeric) and fresh herbs (eg basil, oregano, and garlic) are anti-inflammatory, anti-microbial, and immune-boosting.

Spices such as cinnamon can also help to regulate insulin.

Green tea

Green tea can suppress enzymes and androgens involved in acne formation. It's also anti-inflammatory.

Walnuts/almonds

These nuts might help with blood/skin fatty acid status, and control blood sugar. Monounsaturated fats can be anti-microbial.

Dark green & purple vegetables/fruits

These contain acne fighting anti-oxidants and minerals that extinguish inflammation. They may also inhibit androgen-forming and acne-promoting enzymes.

Free-range organic (or pastured) eggs

Hens that receive nutritious feed (or even better, free-ranging pasture that includes bugs and other small animals) produce more nutrient-dense eggs (including beneficial vitamin A and omega-3 fatty acids) that may help to deter acne.

Tomatoes

These may lower IGF-1 in the body.

Resveratrol

Found in grapes, red wine, peanuts and mulberries.

Vitamin B5 (pantothenic acid)

Supplementation with pantothenic acid (500-1000 mg daily should be sufficient) can be quite effective, and a far safer alternative to commercial prescription medications such as oral contraceptives and retinoids.

Zinc & selenium

6% of all zinc found in our bodies is in our skin. Selenium is a potent antioxidant. It's best to get these in food format.

High-zinc foods include seafood, wild game, red meat, nuts, seeds, and mushrooms. High-selenium foods include nuts (Brazil nuts in particular), fish, poultry, meat, wild game, mushrooms, whole grains, and eggs.

Who doesn't get acne?

Observing cultural shifts in diet can also clue us into what foods might be associated with acne.

Acne doesn't seem to appear in non-Westernized populations eating traditional diets. This includes Inuit, Okinawa islanders, Ache hunter-gatherers, Kitavan islanders, and rural villages in Kenya, Zambia and Bantu.

Staple foods among cultures where acne is nearly absent include:

Tubers (e.g. taro, yam)

Fruit

Fish, seafood, and marine mammals

Coconut

Vegetables

Wild game

Groundnuts and tree nuts

Traditionally prepared (fermented or ash-treated) non-wheat grains such as millet, barley, maize (corn), or rice

Beneficial fungi, molds, and lichen

They don't eat processed foods, sugars, flours or processed wheat, processed oils, nor much dairy. They also get plenty of vitamin D from being outside, and/or consuming the livers of marine animals.

Acne is complex, and each person is unique. However, there are common factors in cultures that don't suffer from acne.

They eat whole, unprocessed foods. All their nutrients come from these foods. They don't supplement.

They get outside and get sunlight (or, again, consume vitamin D in organ meats).

They often eat fermented foods — foods that are high in beneficial probiotics for gut health.

Except for the Inuit, they eat a lot of unprocessed and/or traditionally prepared plant foods, such as fresh or fermented vegetables and fruits, and grains that are soaked/sprouted/fermented.

They often eat many fresh herbs and spices, as well as beneficial fungi. They eat a good balance of unprocessed fats. They eat plenty of omega-3 fatty acids from fish, wild game, and even insects and snails. They don't consume a lot of omega-6s from vegetable or seed oils.

They eat traditionally prepared ground nuts (e.g. peanuts) and tree nuts (e.g. walnuts, almonds).

They don't consume much dairy. If they do, it's fermented and/or pastured.

They eat as much as possible of any animals consumed: dark and white meat, organ meats, connective tissues, etc.

Experiment for yourself

If you struggle with acne, keep a food diary. Look for connections between foods and breakouts — and don't forget that it might take a day or more for foods to stimulate breakouts.

One good experiment is to try doing without wheat, dairy, and sugar for a month to see if it helps. These foods have the strongest associations with acne. Substitute tubers, fruit, and beans/legumes for carbohydrate instead. If that seems like too much, try just one thing at a time.

Other factors

During times of hormonal fluctuation (like puberty) excess sebum production likely occurs to protect hair follicle growth.

Our skin is replaced every 28 to 45 days. Sebaceous glands have receptors for neuropeptides, like endorphins.

Histamines and anti-histamines may influence sebaceous gland function.

Environmental pollutants might bump up IGF-1 levels. Pollution — which includes smoking — also increases oxidation. Smoking can also influence acetylcholine, and acetylcholine can influence sebaceous gland activity.

Natural topical treatments

The plant extracts from Azadirachta indica (Neem), Sphaeranthus indicus (Hindi), Hemidesmus indicus (Sarsaparilla), Rubia cordifolia (Common Madder) and Curcuma longa (Turmeric) seem to be anti-inflammatory and might suppress bacteria on the skin that promote acne. Same with topical tea tree oil.

If you're looking for a cheap vitamin A cream, try egg yolk. Dab it on your skin and leave it for 10 minutes or even overnight (just remember to wash it off eventually).

Chamomile and peppermint tea can soothe skin irritation. Make a strong solution of chamomile and peppermint, swish your face in it, and let it sit for a while on the skin. Plain oatmeal will also calm skin down (again, wash it off eventually unless you're auditioning for a zombie movie).

Fruit acids and enzymes can give you a natural "glycolic peel". Next time you throw fruit in your smoothie, wipe your face with the pineapple or squished orange rinds. Seriously. Plain yogurt also works as a topical probiotic and exfoliating acid.

7
TREATMENTS AND DRUGS

If over the counter (non-prescription) products haven't cleared up your acne, your doctor can prescribe stronger medications or other therapies. A dermatologist can help you:

Control your acne

Avoid scarring or other damage to your skin

Make scars less noticeable

Acne medications work by reducing oil production, speeding up skin cell turnover, fighting bacterial infection or reducing inflammation — which helps prevent scarring. With most prescription acne drugs, you may not see results for four to eight weeks, and your skin may get worse before it gets better. It can take many months or years for your acne to clear up completely.

The drug your doctor recommends depends on the type and severity of your acne. It might be something you apply to your skin (topical medication) or take by mouth (oral medication). Often, drugs are used in combination. Pregnant women will not be able to use oral prescription medications for acne.

Talk with your doctor about the risks and benefits of medications and other treatments you are considering.

Topical medications

These products work best when applied to clean, dry skin about 15 minutes after washing. You may not see the benefit of this treatment for a few weeks. And you may notice skin irritation at first, such as redness, dryness and peeling.

Your doctor may recommend steps to minimize these side effects, including using a gradually increased dose, washing off the medication after a short application or switching to another medication.

The most common topical prescription medications for acne are:

Retinoid: These come as creams, gels and lotions. Retinoid drugs are derived from vitamin A and include tretinoin (Avita, Retin-A, others), adapalene (Differin) and tazarotene (Tazorac, Avage). You apply this medication in the evening, beginning with three times a week, then daily as your skin becomes used to it. It works by preventing plugging of the hair follicles.

Antibiotics: These work by killing excess skin bacteria and reducing redness. For the first few months of treatment, you may use both a retinoid and an antibiotic, with the antibiotic applied in the morning and the retinoid in the evening. The antibiotics are often combined with benzoyl peroxide to reduce the likelihood of developing antibiotic resistance. Examples include clindamycin with benzoyl peroxide (Benzaclin, Duac, Acanya) and erythromycin with benzoyl peroxide (Benzamycin).

Dapsone (Aczone): This gel is most effective when combined with a topical retinoid. Skin side effects include redness and dryness.

Oral medications

Antibiotics. For moderate to severe acne, you may need oral antibiotics to reduce bacteria and fight inflammation. Choices for treating acne include tetracyclines, such as minocycline and doxycycline.

Your doctor will probably recommend tapering off these

medications as soon as your symptoms begin to improve or as soon as it becomes clear the drugs aren't helping — usually, within three to four months. Tapering helps prevent antibiotic resistance by minimizing undue exposure to these medications over a long time.

You will likely use topical medications and oral antibiotics together. Studies have found that using topical benzoyl peroxide along with oral antibiotics may reduce the risk of developing antibiotic resistance.

Antibiotics may cause side effects, such as an upset stomach and dizziness. These drugs also increase your skin's sun sensitivity. They can cause discoloration of developing teeth and reduced bone growth in children born to women who took tetracyclines while pregnant.

The most common side effects of these drugs are headache, breast tenderness, nausea, weight gain and breakthrough bleeding. A serious potential complication is a slightly increased risk of blood clots.

Anti-androgen agent: The drug spironolactone (Aldactone) may be considered for women and adolescent girls if oral antibiotics aren't helping. It works by blocking the effect of androgen hormones on the sebaceous glands. Possible side effects include breast tenderness, painful periods and the retention of potassium.

Isotretinoin: This medicine is reserved for people with the most severe acne. Isotretinoin (Amnesteem, Claravis, Sotret) is a powerful drug for people whose acne doesn't respond to other treatments.

Oral isotretinoin is very effective. But because of its potential side effects, doctors need to closely monitor anyone they treat with this drug. The most serious potential side effects include ulcerative colitis, an increased risk of depression and suicide, and severe birth defects.

In fact, isotretinoin carries such serious risk of side effects that women of reproductive age in the US must participate in a Food and Drug Administration-approved monitoring program to receive a prescription for the drug.

Therapies

These therapies may be suggested in select cases, either alone or in combination with medications.

Light therapy. A variety of light-based therapies have been tried with success. But further study is needed to determine the ideal method, light source and dose.

Light therapy targets the bacteria that cause acne inflammation. Some types of light therapy are done in a doctor's office. Blue-light therapy can be done at home with a hand-held device.

Possible side effects of light therapy include pain, temporary redness and sensitivity to sunlight.

Chemical peel. This procedure uses repeated applications of a chemical solution, such as salicylic acid. It is most effective when combined with other acne treatments, except oral retinoids. Chemical peels aren't recommended for people taking oral retinoids because together these treatments can significantly irritate the skin.

Chemicals peels may cause temporary, severe redness, scaling and blistering, and long-term discoloration of the skin.

Extraction of whiteheads and blackheads. Your dermatologist uses special tools to gently remove whiteheads and blackheads (comedos) that haven't cleared up with topical medications. This technique may cause scarring.

Steroid injection. Nodular and cystic lesions can be treated by injecting a steroid drug directly into them. This improves their appearance without the need for extraction. The side effects of this technique include thinning of the skin, lighter skin and the appearance of small blood vessels on the treated area.

Treating acne scars

Procedures used to diminish scars left by acne include:

Soft tissue fillers. Injecting soft tissue fillers, such as collagen or fat, under the skin and into indented scars can fill out or stretch the skin. This makes the scars less noticeable.

Results are temporary, so you would need to repeat the injections periodically. Side effects include temporary swelling, redness and bruising.

Chemical peels. High-potency acid is applied to your skin to remove the top layer and minimize deeper scars.

Dermabrasion. This procedure is usually reserved for more severe scarring. It involves sanding (planing) the surface layer of skin with a rotating brush. This helps blend acne scars into the surrounding skin.

Laser resurfacing. This is a skin resurfacing procedure that uses a laser to improve the appearance of your skin.

Light therapy. Certain lasers, pulsed light sources and radiofrequency devices that don't injure the epidermis can be used to treat scars. These treatments heat the dermis and cause new skin to form.

After several treatments, acne scars may appear less noticeable. This treatment has shorter recovery times than some other methods. But you may need to repeat the procedure more often and results are subtle.

Skin surgery. Using a minor procedure called punch excision, your doctor cuts out individual acne scars and repairs the hole at the scar site with stitches or a skin graft.

Treating children

Most studies of acne drugs have involved people 12 years of age or older. Increasingly, younger children are getting acne as well.

In one study of 365 girls ages 9 to 10, 78% of them had acne lesions. If your child has acne, you may want to consult a pediatric dermatologist. Ask about drugs to avoid in children, appropriate doses, drug interactions, side effects, and how treatment may affect a child's growth and development.

Treatment of children with acne is often complicated by their family situation. For example, if a child moves between two homes due to divorced parents, it may help to use two sets of medications, one in each home.

8
SKIN CONDITIONS THAT LOOKS LIKE ACNE

In order to correct an aggravating skin condition, you first have to know exactly the problem you are addressing. Many skin problems can be falsely identified as acne, making it difficult, if not impossible to treat. Here are a few common wrongly identified skin conditions.

Folliculitis

This skin condition called Malassezia folliculitis, formerly known as Pityrosporum folliculitis. It is caused by yeasts (fungi) of the genus Malasseziathat which can look just like acne. It looks like small, non-inflamed bumps that frequently shows up on the forehead, but can be anywhere on the face or body.

Folliculitis occurs when bacteria or fungi enters and infect a hair follicle, resulting in inflammation. The inflammation shows up on the skin as a red, sometimes itchy rash of raised bumps. Some people think these bumps are acne, but it's not the same thing.

Most of the time the pores are only filled with a clear liquid instead of pus. It can remain dormant for long periods of time and then flare up with humid weather. This is a good indication that is folliculitis and not acne.

How to treat folliculitis:

Cleansers and serums containing Mandelic acid are great anti-fungal remedies.

Keep the affected areas dry. If it happens on the body use Gold Bond Powder to absorb extra moisture.

Avoid sugar and yeast containing foods such as bread, alcohol, processed/frozen foods, sandwich meat and dairy.

Cotton clothing and cotton sheets are recommended. Avoid using fabric softener and dryer sheets.

Antifungal and probiotic supplements can help heal your digestive system.

Perioral Dermatitis

This skin problem is concentrated around the nose, mouth and chin area, where very small papules and pustules are found. Good indicators that what you have is not acne are that it will become more aggravated with typical acne treatments like exfoliators and benzoyl peroxide.

The affected area tends to be itchy and more closely resembles a rash.

Causes of Perioral Dermatitis are very uncertain however the theories out there are that it is caused by:

Chloride and fluoride found in dental products

Steroid facial creams

Hormones

Sun exposure

Heavy creams and oils

Cold and sun exposure

Oral antibiotics can be an option in severe cases but even then it can reoccur. Some other treatment options include topical antibacterial prescriptions, anti-fungal creams, mild cortisone creams for short-term use.

If you have an outbreak try to avoid the following:

Acne treatment products

Harsh exfoliating products

Cleansers with sulfates and foaming agents

Products with sodium lauryl sulfate

Strawberries, tomatoes, oranges

Chemical sunscreens

Using water based hydrating gel and taking Evening Primrose Oil as a natural supplement can help heal the skin and reduce the dermatitis.

Staph Infections

Staph infections do look much like acne. They are, however, very different, and need proper treatment quickly.

The appearance will differ from acne because they will not have symmetrical edges the way acne does. It could show up as pimples, boils, pus filled lesions, swelling, redness and the skin can feel hot to the touch. This is a serious skin condition and requiring antibiotics to clear.

Staph infections will not improve with acne products and needs to be treated by a physician immediately!

Sebaceous Hyperplasia

This common condition is caused, essentially, by aging skin. Around age 30 androgen levels drop and the skin's cell turnover rate slows down. This can cause a buildup of sebocytes (the cells that make up the oil glands, and secrete sebum) in the sebaceous gland. This decrease in cellular turnover results in a benign enlargement of the sebaceous gland, or sebaceous hyperplasia.

They appear as small donut shaped, skin colored or whitish-yellow small bumps. They can be big or small, and are often found on the face.

When you try to extract them there is no oil coming out because there is no pore opening. They can be removed with electrolysis but the results are not always permanent. Other treatment such as photodynamic therapy, cryotherapy (liquid nitrogen), cau electrodesiccation, topical chemical treatment and laser treatment can help reduce these oil filled bumps.

Pyoderma Faciale

Pyoderma Faciale is much less common, as it can only appear in people who have a particular enzyme deficiency. It does still look much like acne, but it will only be found in the center of the face, while the rest will remain clear. It also generally occurs in women in their 20s and 30s and will be larger and more painful lesions than acne tends to produce.

Brought on by extreme stress or trauma, this will also be accompanied by a severe increase in oil production on the face and in the hair. The condition can be detected from blood samples, and a drug called dexamethasone can slow down testosterone production and reverse the condition.

Steatocystoma Multipex

A rare skin condition, Steatocystoma Multiplex is the presence of many sebum-filled dermal cysts. They will release a gelatinous liquid when you try to extract them, and will fill back up again.

Steatocystoma multiplex is an uncommon disorder of the pilosebaceous unit characterized by the development of numerous sebum-containing dermal cysts.

The relationship of steatocystoma multiplex to the development of sebaceous glands and common presentation at puberty suggest a hormonal trigger for lesion growth.

This is a very difficult condition to treat, and most of the time it caused by hormonal imbalance.

9
WHAT TO DO RIGHT NOW
TO FIX YOUR ACNE

Standby. There's some tough love to finish this book.

It might not make me popular. But I'm hoping it makes your skin better.

By this point in the book you will be thinking one of two things. Either – "Yeah, there was some interesting, useful stuff there."

Or: "I knew all of that."

If it was the former, great. The chances are you will already have formulated the plan you need to make some progress.

Remember that the chances are things won't improve for you immediately or with the first plan of attack you hit upon.

That's OK. It's normal.

Keep going – work through this book little by little and you *will* get there.

But if you have finished reading through and think, "there's nothing there I don't know about" then here is your issue.

(Tough love klaxon!)

You already know what you need to do. But something is stopping you doing it.

It is staggeringly unlikely that none of these suggestions, interventions, lifestyle changes or drugs will work for you.

It is more likely that you feel that you can not ask your doctor for help for some reason. Or you do not want to. Or you are embarrassed. Or you feel you will waste his/her time.

Stop thinking like that.

That is what is holding you back now. Not your spots.

Stop overthinking it. Pick up the phone and make an appointment to see someone.

If this sounds harsh then I'm not sorry for it.

You bought this book to make a change – and I'm running out of pages to help.

So. Whatever you do next – good luck. Things can and will get better for you. And probably sooner than you think.

This does not go on forever.

And no matter what your acne has tried to teach you... you are in control.

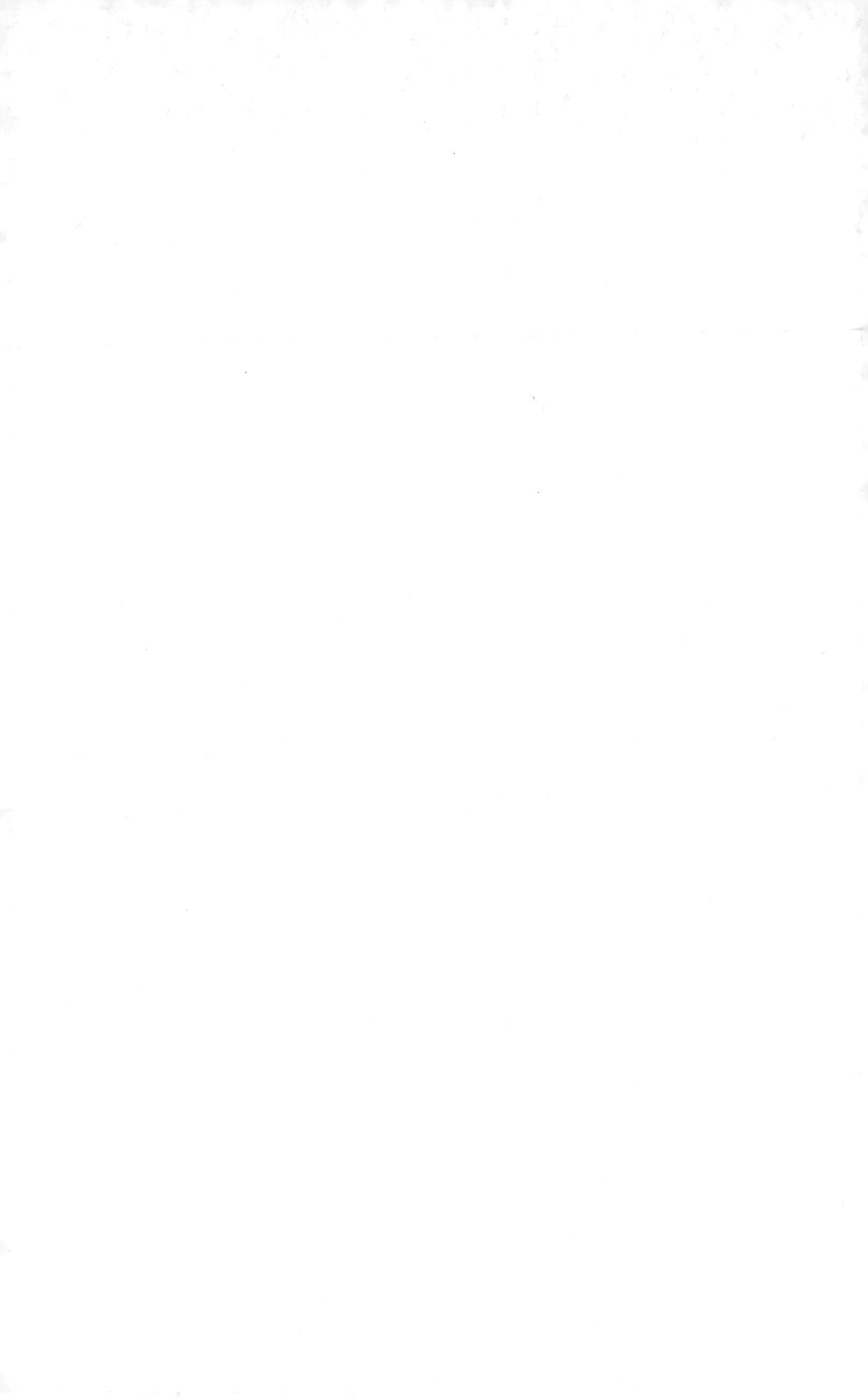